CW00373385

A Handbook For Pagan Healers

Liz Joan

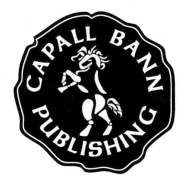

A Handbook For Pagan Healers

ISBN 186163 0336

ALL RIGHTS RESERVED

Photographs by Clive Seymour
Illustrations of elements and images of the Goddess and God by Jack Gale
Cover design by Paul Mason

Published by:

Capall Bann Publishing
Freshfields
Chieveley
Berks
RG20 8TF

Contents

Acknowledgements

My thanks go to Jack, Jon and Julia for believing that I could write this book; to Helen Stirling-Lane for putting it on disc (due to my own computer illiteracy); to Jack Gale for his drawings of the Elementals and images of the Goddess and God; to Clive Seymour for his photographs which add an extra dimension to this book; to Mark for trying to teach me how to use the computer. To all of them for their love and support and also to my many other helpers on my journey but most of all to the Goddess and the God for their Presence in my life. Many thanks, much love, Blessed Be!

Introduction

Do we need another book about healing? Many pagans practise healing as part of their usual rituals, surely they don t need another book to explain how to do it? When I put my hands on another person, they get hot and the other person feels better, surely that is all healing is, isn't it? Healing comes naturally to some special people but not everybody is a natural healer, are they?

The answer to these questions are both affirmative and negative. Many of the books already written about healing are not written by practising Pagan healers but by healers with a Christian orientation. This is fine for them, but not as useful for a witch, druid or magician as a book especially from the pagan viewpoint. Yes, healing is a normal activity but it is always possible to improve upon our human abilities, to fine tune them perhaps. Yes, warmth is often a sign that energy is moving, but which way? Are you taking the sickness from the other person? This is not impossible, in fact, it is quite likely that you will feel depleted later.

Healing is natural to many people but it can also be learned as a skill. There are born artists and musicians but many others can also draw or learn to play an instrument! Healing is an art which anybody can learn and use to benefit friends, family, animals and plants. As more people begin to develop this healing potential, the impact for good on our world could be transformational.

So who am I to write this book? My life started during World War 2 and for my safety I was evacuated to a village in Herefordshire near the Welsh borders. My early care was shared between my mother, an older local woman and her husband who was a gardener at the big house.

For hours I was put in my pram near Uncle Tom who talked to me about his work, why some things grew better in certain places, how to care for the plants and especially how to gain co-operation from the bees. (He was also a bee keeper!) His wife taught my mother how to use traditional remedies and when at 2 years of age I was seriously ill with whooping cough I was treated with honey, lemon and glycerine, lots of fresh air and cuddles! The same treatment worked well for my own child over 20 years later!

Without realising what I was doing I used healing throughout my life as a nursery teacher, tending small wounds, pacifying distressed children and worried parents. Later when learning massage I encountered the hot hands situation and decided to learn all I could about this energy exchange which was taking place. I studied for a Diploma in Healing with The College of Healing in Malvern, Worcestershire and re-visited my early home a few miles away in Hereford. I also encountered and was attuned to Reiki whilst studying with the College and completed a Diploma in Counselling. Currently I teach an Introduction to

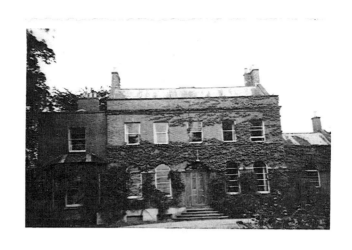

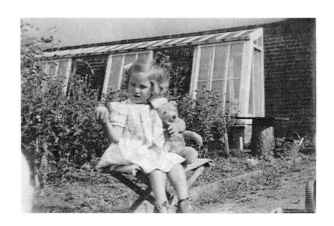

Top: Sutton Court, the author's early childhood home
Bottom: Liz, aged 2 in Sutton Court garden

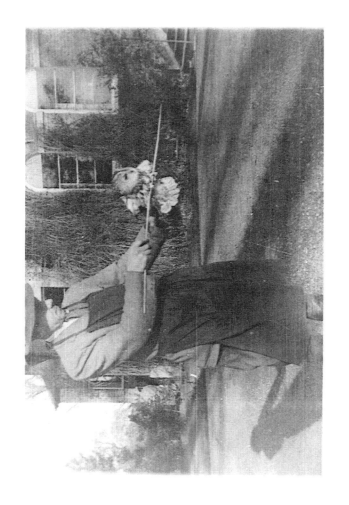

Uncle Tom with a young owl (1941)

Healing course run by The College of Healing and am a Reiki master and a witch.

The aim of this book is to provide a working guide for those pagans who wish to develop their healing potential safely and to give practical suggestions as to how this can be done. It is in no way prescriptive - there are many ways to heal - this is my way which I share with you in the hope that you will find it useful. May you have joy as you tread the path of learning and may the Goddess and the God be with you on the journey.

Blessed Be.

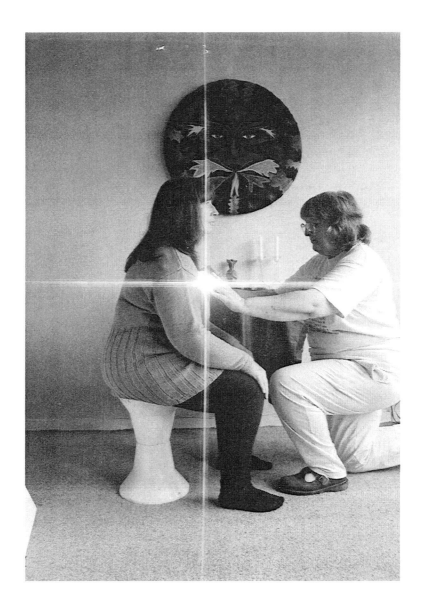

Chapter 1

What is Healing?

To answer this question we must first define health. The dictionary says Health is the state of an organism functioning normally without disease or abnormality. A state of optimal functioning, well-being or progress. Most important is the aspect of disease - a word which can be split into its component parts - dis-ease. So we have a double negative with *absence* and *dis* giving us the understanding that health equates with ease . An organism or person at ease with itself is healthy. In order for ease to be that state, the organism or person has to be in a balanced condition. So, balance = ease = health. When a person or organism is balanced, at ease or healthy, then it is in a state of well-being and optimal functioning. Healing is the action or effect which creates health and the healer is the tool by which this happens. Looking now at the organism, be it person, animal, plant or any other being which is made of energy, there are many different levels of that being which may be at dis-ease within themselves or with other levels within the organism, so healing needs to be directed to the appropriate level, be it physical or etheric.

This brings us to awareness of the aura which is part of each of us. Everyday phrases like " you're crowding me" or " he's in my space" acknowledge that we are often aware of another person' s energy field intruding or overlapping with our own. When working in a circle this energy is combined and enhanced by sound and/or movement when raising a Cone of Power.

Within any working group, the group energy is important and this is something more than personal interactions or friendships. I shall make further reference to this group energy when discussing absent or distant healing.

The aura has many levels but those which are most often affected by disease are the mental and emotional levels (or subtle bodies). These can be felt with practice, as hot or cold areas around the physical body and healing energy can be directed to these areas to restore balance and wholeness. Each level or body within the aura is linked to a chakra or energy centre.

The word *chakra* in Sanskrit means 'wheel'. These spinning vortexes of energy are like gateways into the appropriate subtle body of the person. For the organism to be in balance it is necessary for the chakras to be clear and balanced. It is possible, and in fact essential, to be able to open and close our own chakras at will and this is what we do when we open up or attune to each other and the Goddess/God or when we close down , open the circle or end the rite.

The Base or Root chakra is at the base of the spine. It connects with and absorbs energy from the earth and is concerned with the base instinctual will to survive. It is seen as red and the conditions which it helps to balance are those related to the physical structure of the body, i.e. skeleton and muscular systems, especially those in the feet or legs. Its ruling planet is Saturn and its element is earth.

The Sacral chakra is just below the navel. It is concerned with balancing the lower digestive system and the reproductive system. It is seen as orange and relates to basic emotions, creativity and sexuality. Any blocked energy in this chakra may be caused by the person having no outlet for his/her creative energies and if the Throat chakra is also not functioning fully he/she will not be able to express the need for creativity. The Sacral chakra is ruled by the moon and its related element is water.

The Solar Plexus chakra is at the base of the sternum or breastbone and it is concerned with the upper digestive system including the stomach and with the emotions. It also relates to the autonomic nervous system. When a person is "sick with fear" or gets "butterflies" when under stress it is this chakra which needs balancing and healing. The Solar Plexus is seen as yellow. Its element is fire and its ruling planet is Mars.

The Heart chakra is in the centre of the sternum and it is seen as green. It relates to the higher emotions of love and compassion. On a physical level it is concerned with the heart, circulatory system and lungs. The Heart chakra is ruled by the planet Venus and its element is air.

The Throat chakra is found at the throat! It is concerned with self-expression and communication. It maintains balance in the upper chest and throat including the speech organs. It is seen as blue and is ruled by the planet Mercury. Its element is ether.

The Brow or Third Eye chakra is in the centre of the forehead. It relates to the pituitary gland-the mother gland of the endocrine system and is concerned with intuition, clairvoyance and high sense perception. It is seen as indigo blue, it is ruled by the planet Jupiter and its element is thought.

The Crown chakra is situated on the top of the head and is our link to the Cosmic forces and Goddess/God energy. The central nervous system is controlled by this chakra as the brain and spinal cord are an important part of this system. It is seen as violet or white and is ruled by the planet Uranus. The element related to the Crown chakra is light.

So healing is the process by which the healer brings balance and ease to the healee at all levels of her/his being. The healer is bringing about change by the power of her/his mind, focusing the healing energy by application of will and intent. The process of healing IS a magical process and by invoking the powers of the Universe to help the self-healing process of the healee, the healer is in the role of Priest or Priestess.

In his article *Magic for Healing - a Shamanic Perspective* in *Chaos International* No.21, Phil Hine states that healing is an aspect of sorcery. Certainly during times of persecution the healer has been at risk and many of the aspects of the Pagan path are also aspects of healing. The study of herbs, of crystals, of aromatic oils and incense are some of these aspects which are worthy of further investigation for the Pagan healer because they are all part of the knowledge of the Wise woman/healer and are all components in the wider complementary medicine field which includes healing.

The village wise woman or tribal shaman knew which plants would be useful in certain times of life or to help dis-ease; they also knew which places or which rocks were helpful when meditating or needing healing of the spirit - this is using the energy from the earth in much the same way as crystals can be used. From very early times we know that oils and incenses were used to promote feelings of well-being and altered states of consciousness. In ancient cultures the work of healing was part of the role of the priest or priestess working within a sacred space. This is still the case for those of us who work as priests, priestesses, druids or magicians. We may sometimes need to create sacred space in the home or hospital of our patients but the work is the same.

One misconception which I feel must be corrected at this stage is that healing a person means that they should then get better, the symptoms should ease and they will recover from the illness. Healing is NOT the same as curing. It is possible that the illness of a patient is part of the learning or development for that person; it may be that it is the right time for this current life to end. The healer offers the healing energy to the spirit of the patient for that person to use in their own best interests. This may mean that the patient accepts the situation, becomes more peaceful and may be able to die and move on with less trauma.

It may also mean that the symptoms do become less and a full recovery will be made! Magic is the process by which we effect change by the application of will and intent. We cannot always be certain what the precise change will be, except that it will be for the good of the patient and this has to be always our reason for offering healing.

There is no need for the patient to consciously believe in any deity or even have any faith in the healer. We are working with the Higher Self or spirit of the patient and this is beyond consciousness or belief systems. As the healer, we intend that the patient will benefit from healing, we do not specify how or when that benefit will occur and do not look to be regarded as the Source of healing, only as the channel through which the healing energy flows. We are like petrol pumps at a service station forecourt, the tank of fuel lies beneath the tarmac and the hose which connects to each vehicle is like our hands on a patient.

Healing is not curing but it is the offering of Earth and Cosmic energy to the Spirit of the patient for their Highest Good. We work as priests or priestesses within a sacred space always focusing on the best interests of our patients and applying our will and intent to that end.

For me, healing is truly working magic and not something to be undertaken lightly. It is doing the work of the Goddess and the God.

Chapter 2

Ethics of Healing

Do healers need an ethical code? The energy can only do good so why bother with ethics, isn't that making it all too intellectual?

If we take our work seriously as befits a magical activity in which the healer is the priest or priestess through whom the Goddess or God energy can flow, then we do need to have ethics and to learn all we can to enable the healing we offer to be appropriate to our clients. In order to learn about healing and to have opportunities to practice in a controlled environment it has often been difficult for pagans as many of the organisations which offer training are Christian spiritualist biased.

There are a few which claim to be non-denominational or non-sectarian but in my experience even these tend to be based on Christian spirituality. I have been fortunate to find training with the College of Healing at Runnings Park in Worcestershire where I have been fully accepted as a witch alongside fellow students who include Quakers, C. of E. Christians, atheists and Druids. Courses in healing, meditation, channelling and magic are also run at the same venue giving it an aura of acceptability to all religions, paganism included. As the College is a member of the Confederation of Healing Organisations (C.H.O.), all members of the college (M.C.O.H.) are bound by the code of conduct of the C.H.O. which among other requirements states that public liability and professional indemnity insurance is mandatory. If you are working as a healer professionally this is exactly what you need as a complementary therapist but if you are only working occasionally with a few friends then you will not need a professional qualification or insurance. For this situation, a course like the Introduction to Healing course offered by the college or similar training at the College of Psychic Studies or some other organisation would be much more appropriate.

Wherever you do your further learning about developing the ability to channel healing energy you will find that certain basic rules for ethics will apply.

1. Nobody can be made to accept healing and it is not suggested that 'You look as though you need healing!' is a very good approach! Healing can be offered, allowing the other person to decline if they so wish and always without judgement. Sometimes the physical, conscious body requests healing but the Higher Self or super-conscious may not feel that it is appropriate at that time.

2. All clients must be treated with respect and no judgement should be made regarding the

state of health, religious belief, sexuality, appearance or any other aspect of the client.

3. No healer will physically touch a client without permission from the client and most healing is offered in the aura. If touch is approved by the client such hands-on work would not involve sexually explicit areas of the body.

4. All payment or exchange if appropriate will be agreed before the healing. Many healers will work for donations or no charge at all

5. Healing is offered in good faith by the healer but he/she cannot guarantee what may result and although symptoms may be relieved, healing is not the same thing as curing.

6. No healer is allowed, by law, to give diagnosis of illness. Only a doctor is allowed to diagnose.

All this may sound very structured and mundane, but we do live in the mundane world. Just because we are pagans we are not infallible and we need to be aware of legal requirements.

To constructively mis-quote a Biblical saying we need to "Render unto Caesar, the things that are Caesar's but into the Goddess the things that are Hers."

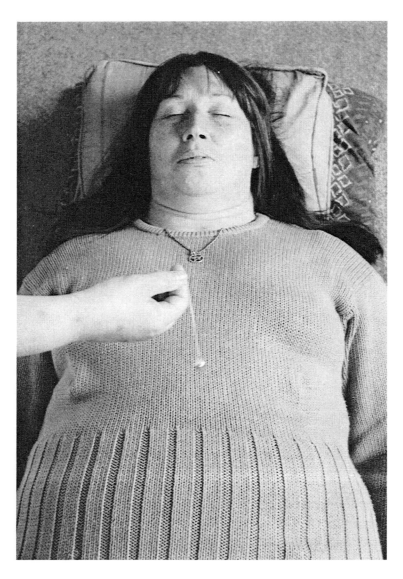

Dowsing and healing the chakras: Method 1

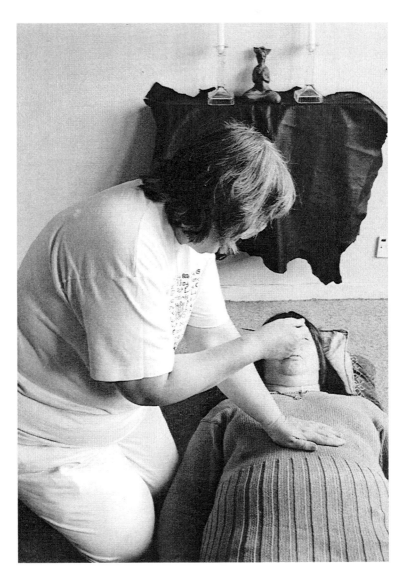

Dowsing and healing the chakras: Method 2

Group preparing for absent healing

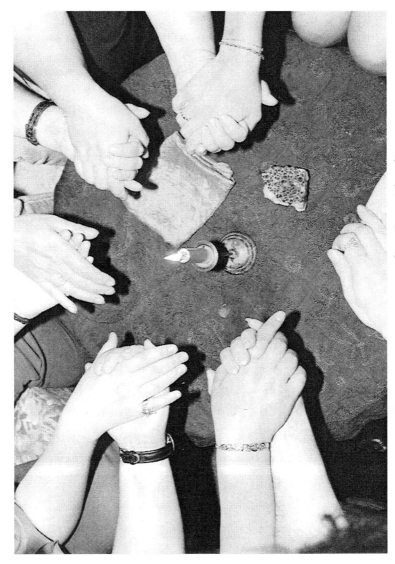

Raising group energy for absent healing

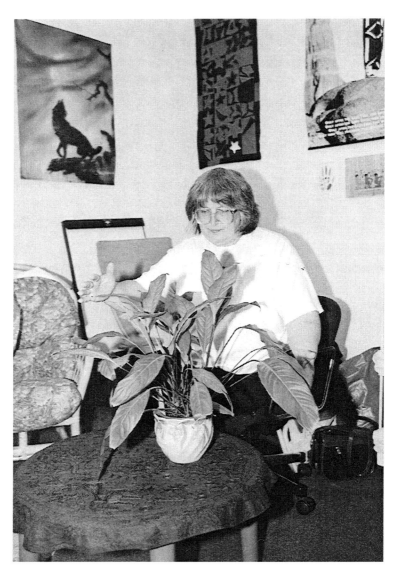

Healing can be given to plants and animals.

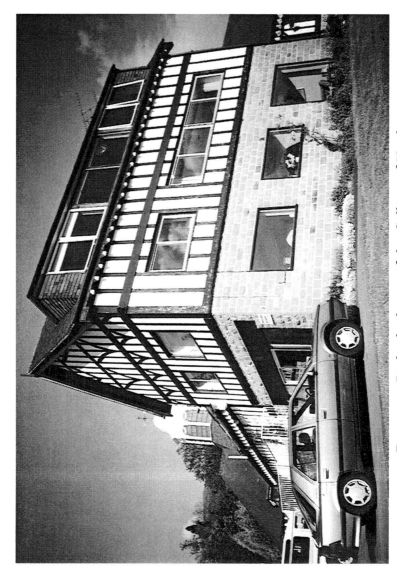

Runnings Park, the home of the College of Healing

Kirlian photography of hands before giving healing (unfocussed energy)

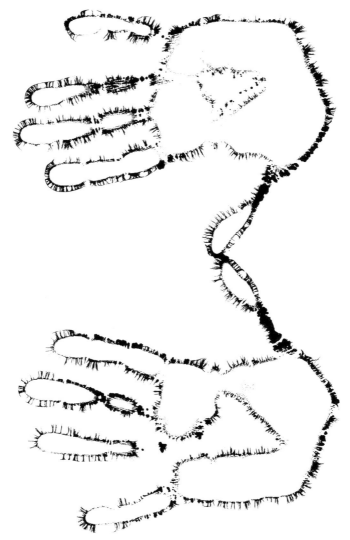

Kirlian photography of hands after giving healing (focused energy)

Chapter 3

Healer, heal thyself

When we offer the healing energy of the Earth and Cosmos to another person, animal or plant we are allowing our body to be used as a channel for that energy. If water is poured through a dirty pipe it comes out of that pipe muddy and contaminated. In the same way if you pipe healing energy through a contaminated vessel it will not be as clear and strong as it would be if the vessel was clean. Some of the energy will have been used to purify the healer. Because of this it is not wise to offer healing if you are unwell unless it is an emergency situation. The energy will still come through but not as clearly as it would normally do. It is also important to remember that disease of the healer may not only be physical but can occur at all levels of our beings.

If we are to work regularly with healing energy then it stands to reason that we need to maintain our own person at optimal fitness. However, nobody is perfect - if we had learnt all the lessons this life has to offer then we would not be here, and one of the lessons we need to learn is to accept our own limitations. The important thing is that we are aware of the areas in our own lives where we could improve and take steps towards that improvement. The areas of life to look at can be summarized into four sections; what we eat, what we drink, what we breath and what we think. What we put in our bodies makes them what they are.

Eating

When we are offering healing we are working with an energy of a very high vibration and if our own body is functioning at a low vibration it can affect the healing. It is advisable to eat light preferably vegetarian meals before giving healing. (Plants have the highest vibratory level of all.) You may like to consider also the quality of the food you eat. Fresh foods which have been grown organically without the use of chemicals are better for the digestive system. Do you really want to eat pesticides and hormonal preparations designed to improve the yield and appearance of your food? If we are caring for our physical body we want to give it the best fuel to work on that we can provide. Mother Earth offers us of her fruits and vegetables - who are we to improve upon Her offering?

Hail and thanks to the Spirits of Earth.

Drinking

Do you drink enough water every day? Around two litres would be about right - not tea, coffee, wine, beer etc but pure clean water. O.K., so the water from the tap is not pure - so use a filter or drink spring water. If you live near a source of spring water then use it, if not buy it bottled. Water helps to keep the body clean inside as well as outside by diluting the toxic effects of cell action or over use of drugs like alcohol or caffeine. It makes the work of the kidneys much easier and so they are less likely to suffer from congestion or overwork. Many reflexologists will testify to the fact that all too many clients have congestion or blocked energy around their kidney points. Drinking plenty of water will both cleanse and refresh the body.

Hail and thanks to the Spirits of Water.

Breathing
We take air into our lungs; we also breathe in all the pollutants in that air which can create dis-ease. The case against cigarette smoking is only one aspect of this. We as pagans need to be concerned too with the air quality of the place where we live and maybe be prepared to support groups who campaign for cleaner air. If we drive a car, we need to be sure that it produces as few pollutants as possible and only to use the vehicle when it is really necessary. A ten minute walk is much healthier for the body and the environment than a two minute drive. It is also good to visit places where the air is clearer and more pleasant to breathe - by the sea-shore or up a hill or mountain perhaps. We need air to survive on this planet, we who honour the Spirits of Air must help to preserve and purify it.

Hail and thanks to the Spirits of Air.

Thinking
When we listen to the News or watch T.V. we are putting something into our bodies which affects how

we think or feel. National or international disasters reported with horrifying pictures or sounds make us feel bad and start our thoughts turning to negative reactions. Why did it have to happen? Couldn't somebody stop this outrage? etc. We do need to be aware of world events but do we need to watch entertainment which is of a horrifying or negative content?

When you are about to give healing through your hands, using your will and intent, that will has to be clear and focused. It does not need to be polluted by negative thoughts or emotions and so it is important that as a healer you monitor what messages and images your brain receives when you are about to give healing in order that your energy can be strong to work for good.

Hail and thanks to the Spirits of Fire, give us of your cleaning, transfiguring energy.

After all these dire warnings (!) what can we do that is positive to help keep ourselves healthy and balanced? Eat well, drink well, breathe well and keep a healthy mind. Take exercise for the body and do meditation for the mind and spirit. If we are allowing the healing of the Goddess and the God to flow through us, then surely it behoves us to provide a fitting vessel to carry the energy. If we de-value the vessel we also de-value the Energy.

Loving Lady and Sweet Lord allow Your Healing Energy to flow through me to those who request it. I will do my best to keep the Vessel clean.

Chapter 4

Protection

Why bother with protecting yourself? If you are giving healing then you are channelling good energy, the Goddess will see that you are safe! So say many healers and to some extent I agree, but the Goddess helps those who help themselves. It is no good putting your hand on a burner on the cooker saying that the Goddess will stop you getting hurt - it doesn't work that way.

We as human beings have an intellectual ability to understand the rule of cause and effect. If you take risks, you may get hurt. To take risks unnecessarily for no good reason other than that you can't be bothered, is both stupid and not worthy of an image of the Goddess or the God which ever you are.

So why can healing be a risk-taking activity? If we remember that the client is suffering from dis-ease or ill-ness then we are aware that negative feelings or energies may be present in that person. In order that the healer does not allow these energies to transfer back into him/herself a barrier is needed between them. I hear the question - how can you offer healing through a barrier? Very easily if the barrier is so programmed that only positive energies can pass through it!

Accepting that some form of protection for the healer is needed we then have to decide on what form this will take. We are working with energies and in order to take care of ourselves and to work efficiently with these energies the healer needs to have developed the ability to visualise light, colours and shapes at will. This is not as difficult as it may seem and when you spend a few minutes daily in meditation and practise your visualisations regularly they will begin to come when you call them up.

The quickest and simplest and in my experience the most efficient protection is to use gold, blue, white or silver light (depending on your colour preference!) in a circular shape, either linear or spherical, again depending on your personal preference. This may sound familiar to many of my readers. Of course it is a magic circle! Why do many of us do our magical work inside a circle cast using visualised light/energy? We do it to provide a sacred place set aside that is safe and protected. When we visualise a sphere or circle of light around ourselves, our clients and our working space we are casting our own circles of power within which we can offer healing safely.

When I offer healing to a person the first circle is cast by visualisation around that person, the second circle is cast around myself and unless I am already working in a cast circle, the third is cast around both the healee and myself. All circles are then programmed by your will to allow healing energy to flow between them and in the case of the healee to allow negative energies to flow out away from him/her. When the outer circle is taken down this will flow away into the earth or cosmos to be transformed and cleaned.

After finishing the healing work, it is important to take down the protection set by the healer and to clear the energies in the room. However, it can be very helpful to talk the healee through a very simple self-protection visualisation before they leave and before you clear the room/space. I offer this to my own clients:

> Feel yourself sitting comfortably on the chair. Place your feet flat on the ground and feel your firm connection with the Earth. Allow your body to feel relaxed with your head balanced easily on the top of your spine.
>
> (Allow a few moments quiet)
>
> Focus on your breathing, allow it to become slower and deeper, letting go a little more with each out-breath.
>
> (Allow plenty of time and watch the healee for three breaths)
>
> *Now bring your awareness to your very centre of your being at your solar plexus, below the base of your rib cage. Picture deep inside a tiny candle burning - your life-force, life-spark, and allow the beautiful golden, yellow candle glow to spread throughout your physical body. Feel it spread its light and warmth through your chest and abdomen, down your legs, right down to your toes.*

down your arms to your very fingertips and up your neck to fill your head with its cleansing healing, pure light and energy.

(Allow plenty of time here, speaking gently and slowly. Try to attune to see this happening but don't worry if you just guess when the healee is ready!)

When your physical body is full of light, just allow the energy to flow out into your aura to about 12-15 inches out from your physical body and then let the outside surface become set, firm like the skin inside a bird's egg. Nod when you have pictured this.

(Wait for the nod)

Now put on the outside of the skin whatever feels appropriate, it needs to be strong and may be coloured or armour plated. Whatever it is, it will only allow good energy to come through to you and will protect you from harm.

When you are sure that your egg-shaped protection is in place, bring your awareness back into the room, the chair on which you are sitting. Open your eyes, stand up and stamp a few times to ground yourself.

With practice, this procedure can be completed in a few minutes and may be repeated wherever it feels necessary.

If you are going to work as a healer, or if you already do so, then it is important to practise the visualisation needed for protection. Using this method you will not pick up the symptoms of your clients nor will you give them anything other than the pure healing energy of the Earth or Cosmos, Goddess or God.

Chapter 5

Meditation: a few notes

In order to develop the ability to centre oneself and attune to the healing energies it is helpful to practise meditation on a regular basis. This will enable you to centre yourself, set up the relevant protection and attune to the energies quite quickly and easily.

There are many ways to meditate, all of which are valid and allow one to link in to one's own inner space as well as the Goddess and God energy. Often a guided meditation or path working, using another person, tape or book may be useful to help focus inwards but equally valid is to sit in silence and allow space for the Goddess/God to speak to you.

When setting out to meditate there are several aspects which need consideration. Firstly, where will you meditate? The place needs to be quiet with no disturbance, the telephone put on answerphone (if you have one) or ringer turned off, any pets settled elsewhere, no visitors, relatives or children likely to call you and obviously radios and televisions turned off!

Next, how are you going to position yourself? You may wish to lie down but this may be risky if you are tired - you may just fall asleep. If you are sitting it is best to either sit on the floor cross legged or on a chair with feet flat on the floor and hands on your lap. In either case, try to keep your back straight with your head balanced easily on the top of your spine.

Now decide what you want to be the focus of your meditation. Allow your mind to empty of unwanted thoughts, simply let them go, then focus on your chosen subject or turn on your tape player.

After spending time in meditation, it is important that you return fully to your physical body and ground yourself. There are various methods of grounding - eating a little food or stamping your feet are methods which I use and recommend.

You may choose to use a meditation which involves movement. This could be linked to yoga or t'ai chi or may be simply moving to music or a rhythmic beat on a drum.

However you choose to meditate, that way needs to be right for you. The choice is yours but if you take your channelling of Healing energy seriously you will also allow some time each day to hear the voice of the Caring Goddess or Healing God. Listen well!

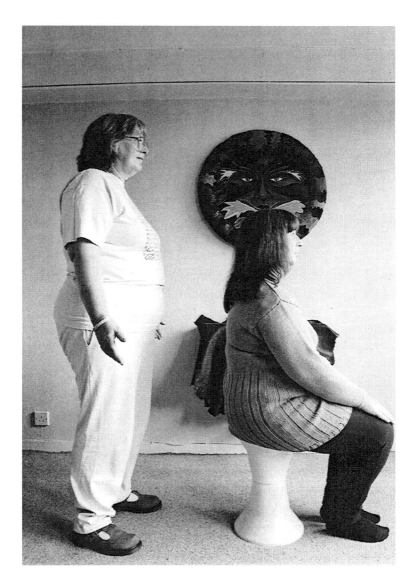

Setting up protection, drawing energy from Earth and Cosmos

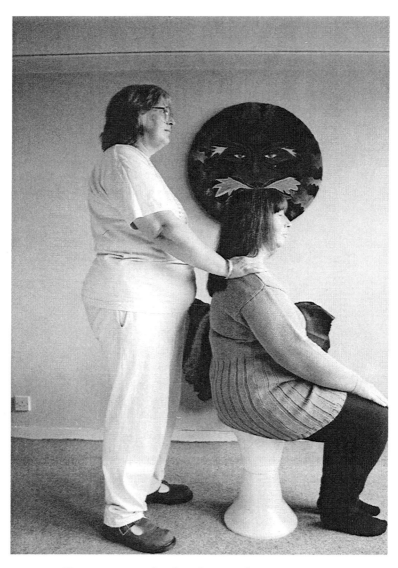

Tuning into the healee, asking permission

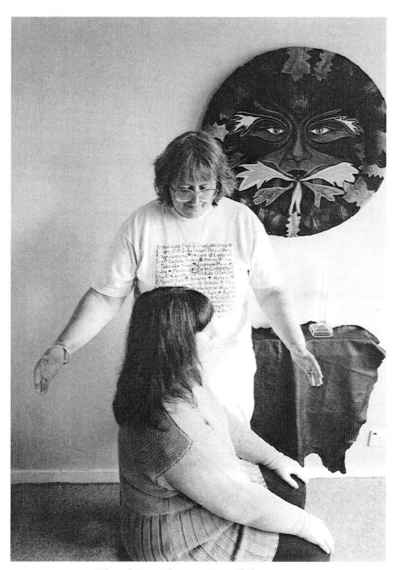

Checking the state of the aura

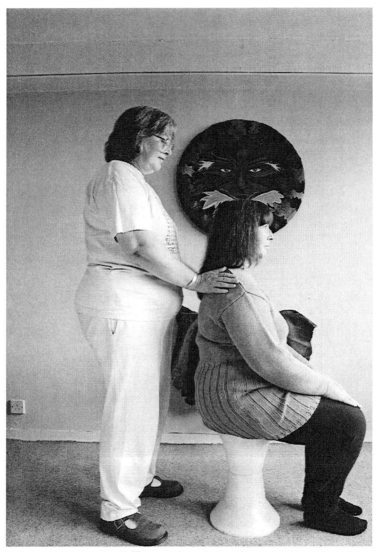

Offering healing energy

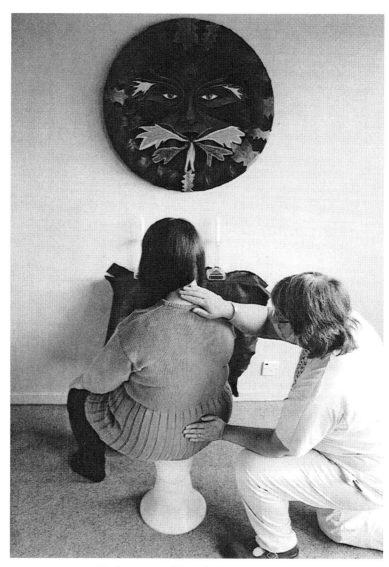

Balancing Kundalini energy

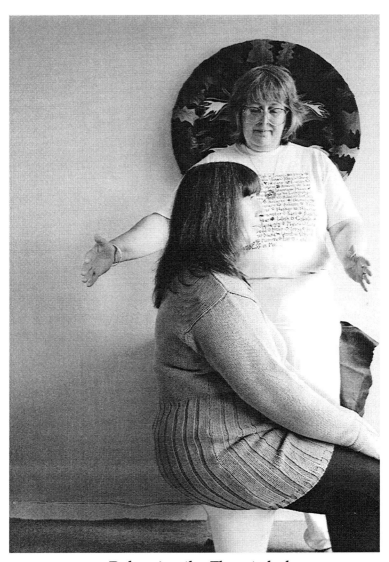

Balancing the Throat chakra

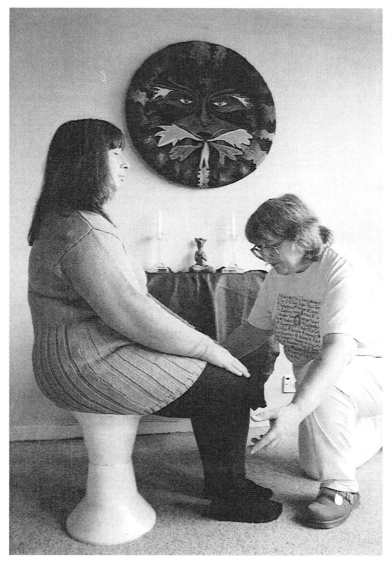

Sieving the aura

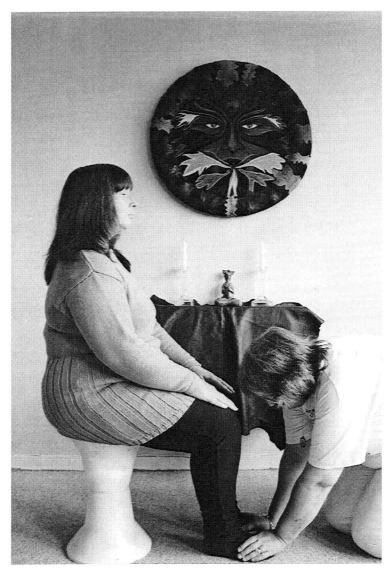

Grounding the healee

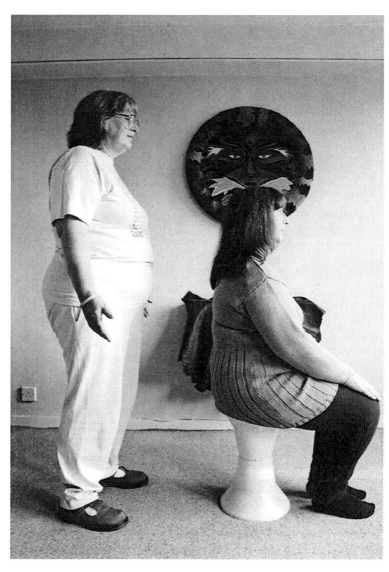

Disconnection, take down protection, thank the Source of Healing

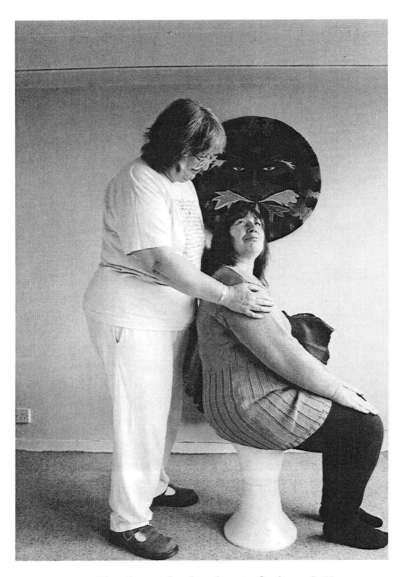

Checking the healee is feeling O.K.

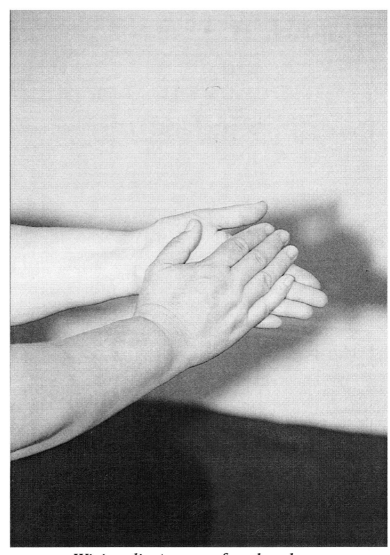

Wiping client energy from hands

Chapter 6

"How to" in easy stages and absent healing

Once other people know that you work within healing energies you will often be asked to give or channel healing. Frequently you will be asked in seemingly inappropriate places, often in pubs, at conferences or parties. When this occurs you will be faced with decisions.

Firstly have you yourself been drinking alcohol and if so, how much? When you are experienced in this healing field, it is possible to channel energy with a small quantity of alcohol in your blood, though it is NOT to be recommended. The energy will not be clear and your own ability to provide you or your client with protection will be impaired. The same applies to any other 'social substances' to which you have been exposed or of which you have partaken.

Secondly, when channelling healing energy in any busy or public place, it is essential to construct a safe working space around yourself and the client. If you have any difficulty doing this, then do not give healing at that time; it would be better to send healing energy absently when you are in a more suitable place.

Assuming that you are going to do some healing work first find a place where it is quiet and you are not likely to be disturbed. You may do this work within a circle or ritual and that is a perfect environment, being private and protected! Having found a place, cleanse it with whatever method you usually use. I use salt, water, fire and incense then visualise the whole room filled with golden light. I walk deosil (clockwise) around the room sprinkling the water with salt in it for water and earth; then I do likewise with charcoal and incense or an incense stick to cleanse with fire and air. Then following my usual protection method (see chapter 4) I allow the golden light to overflow from my aura into the room and fill it with energy. Finally I cast a circle of blue/white light around the room or working space.

Once the space is prepared the healee can be brought in and sat on a straight-backed chair. It is helpful to have a few words together when you can ascertain the problems of the healee and also give him/her re-assurance to help him/her to relax. Some people may like to talk the healee through a body relaxation at this point starting with the feet and working up to the head, mentioning each bodypart and the request to let go of any tensions and allow the body to relax. An alternative method is to focus on the breathing and let go a little more with each exhalation.

When the healee is relaxed, move round to stand behind the chair, allow your own chakras to be open, relax your own body and become aware of your own centre of your being. Now set up protective rings or spheres around yourself and the healee as in Chapter 4.

Place your hands on the shoulders of the healee, synchronise your breathing with his/hers and allow yourself to attune to his/her energy. Take your time over this stage, sending intentions of unconditional love to your healee, encouraging relaxation.

Next, offer healing to the healee in your mind, saying silently; 'I *offer this healing for your highest good*'. If the answer is negative, you may feel heat retreating back up your arms. When offering, you are allowing the Higher Self of the healee to say 'No, thank you' as well as 'Yes, please'. If the answer is negative this is not a rejection of you as a healer. It may be helpful to the conscious self of your healee for you to just check the state of the aura and energy matrix of the body without adding healing. They will feel that you have valued them enough to spend time finding out how they are.

To check the aura, bring your hands away from the person and then slowly bring them in again, feeling the levels with the aura of the different subtle bodies. You can feel how large and expanded the aura is or how much it has contracted. To check the energy matrix, you can put one hand on the top of each limb and one half-way down or at the lowest point and feel for the energy passing between your hands. The same can be done with one hand on the neck and one at the base of the spine.

When you feel that the answer is affirmative, focus on the Earth Goddess energy beneath your feet and draw it up your legs to your base chakra, then up your chakric system to your crown allowing it to fall again to the Earth like a fountain. Now, draw down the Solar energy of the God through your crown chakra, down to meet with the Goddess. You are now like a bridge between Earth and the Cosmos, between Goddess and God so allow this mixed energy to flow from your hands into the body of the healee. This is NOT your own personal energy, you are like the plumbing pipes on a shower, where the hot and cold water is mixed to pour out from the shower head (your hands!) as pleasantly warm.

Now, you can check the state of the aura of your healee. If it is small and contracted you may like to offer energy to build it; if it is large at the head and small at the feet, move it around with your hands until it is evenly spread. If there are cold patches, offer warmth, empty patches or holes may like to be repaired. You may be able to differentiate between the subtle bodies and if one needs strengthening then offer strength!

Next you may feel the chakras and offer appropriately coloured light to each of them. DO NOT attempt to feel or heal either the crown or base chakras, these can usually take care of themselves!

To feel the energy matrix as mentioned previously can be helpful, adding healing energy to boost any part which feels depleted. If the healee has a problem with a specific body part, now is the time to offer healing to that part. If it is somewhere which can be touched without giving offence to the healee, you may want to do so. If you are in any doubt whether to touch or if the problem is in the genital area (and breast area in women) then work in the aura, directing healing where it is needed.

When you feel that the healing is complete for this treatment, gently stroke the aura from either side of the crown chakra, down the body and legs to the feet. Visualise the healee's feet firmly rooted in the Earth and hold them physically with a gentle downward pressure for a few moments.

Return to stand behind the chair, thank the Goddess and the God for the healing energy and allow it to return out of the base and crown chakras. Close your own sacral, solar plexus, heart, throat and brow chakras, check that you are grounded and centred. Step back slightly, disconnecting from the healee, take down the protective rings or spheres. Now, shake or wipe the energy from your hands and touch the healee gently on the shoulders to indicate that the healing has been completed.

It can be useful to spend a little while with the healee at this point. You may like to provide a drink of water and discuss the possibility of the healee learning to protect him/herself as described in Chapter 4. At all times treat your healee with unconditional positive regard and remember that he or she is also a vehicle for the God or Goddess.

When sending healing energy absently, it is always safer to visualise the healee coming to you. To do this, prepare your working space as before then prepare yourself by opening your chakras and drawing energy up from the Earth and down from the Cosmos. Next, holding your hands in front of you about shoulder width apart, picture the recipient of healing between them. Offer the healing for the healee's highest good and allow the energy to flow out of your hands. (A variation is to hold a piece of paper with the name of the healee between your hands). After a while, when it feels right, close down the energy with thanks to the Goddess and the God and close down your chakric system.

It can be useful to use group energy for absent healing. Within a Sacred Circle, when the energy has been raised by dance or chant, it is only necessary to bring the healee into the circle by naming him/her and directing thoughts and intents of love and healing for his/her Highest Good to him/her.

If some people have come together especially to send healing but are not working within a circle of power one way to proceed is as follows. All present sit in a circle and if they wish they may hold hands, although this is not essential. After the leader has talked everybody through the opening of the chakras the energy is drawn into each person and then moved clockwise (deosil) around the group, each person sending out to the left and receiving from the right.

When the energy is moving and building each person visualises a beam of golden energy from their solar plexus chakra building a column of golden healing energy in the centre of the circle. Into this column, those who have requested a healing or for whom the healing has been requested are visualised and named.

Any of the healers working can name healees. When all names have been said the leader talks the group through the visualisation of stopping the flow from the solar plexus and then lifting the column and launching it into the universe, lifting it up to the Sun and the Moon for the healees to receive appropriate healing for their Highest Good. Usual thanks and closing down should follow and it should be ensured that all participants are grounded back in their physical bodies.

Whenever a person is channelling healing energy to benefit others it is important to give the thanks to the Goddess and her Consort and to feel honoured by their Presence in this place and at this time.

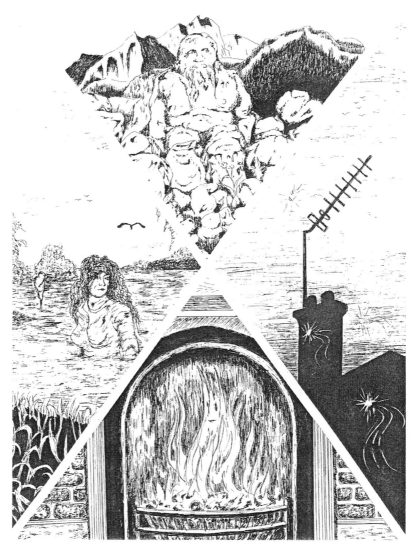

Four Elemental Beings, by Jack Gale

Chapter 7

Using Elemental Energies

Within our understanding of the Universe we accept that there are other realms of existence on other wavelengths or energetic levels not usually visible to the human physical eyes and it is helpful for us to envisage these Realms as being related to the Elements of Earth, Air, Fire and Water in the Western tradition. Again we will often align these Elements with the four main compass directions and we can equate North with Earth elementals, East with Air elementals, South with Fire elementals and the West with Water elementals. When we are involved with channelling healing, having drawn on Goddess and God energy, we can also call on the elementals for their assistance. Certain human conditions can benefit from help from the appropriate Elemental kingdom and it is useful to look at these differing states and how they relate to different Elements.

Earth

The human physical body is the densest of the subtle bodies and so is helped by the energy from the element of Earth. The Earth elementals or gnomes inhabit the rocks, caves, mountains and crystals as well as our own garden soil. In your visualisation you will probably feel drawn to one of these environs and the appearance of the gnome will vary according to where it lives.

Gnomes which I have met have been monochrome brown, appearing to be made up of their Element; they were about three to four feet high, thick set and humanoid with large hands and leathery feet. They appeared to be clothed in rough shirts and trousers and had heavy facial features and neck-length hair. Your perception of a gnome may be very different from mine but what is important is that, if you want to work with the Elemental energies then you do have some perceptions of how these energies appear or feel to you.

The Earth elementals will often be very helpful when working with clients suffering with conditions relating to the skeletal or muscular systems of the body, like arthritis or rheumatism. They can also help with repairing fractures and with problems of the feet. As crystals are of the Earth, the gnomes who inhabit crystal caves and seams in the Earth as are wide in their help as are the crystals themselves. Generally the colour of a crystal will relate to the colour associated with a chakra but if you want to study this aspect of healing there are many good books on the subject.

Air
This element is related to the mental subtle body involved with the thinking, intellectual processes. The

Sylphs of the Air element in my experience are like gentle, transparent floaty shapes or tiny sparks of white or coloured light in the air. As I attempt to focus on them, they float away and appear again on the periphery of my vision. These elusive beings will however always be there if the healer needs assistance when offering healing to a client who has persistent head-aches from stress and overwork or for a person who is thinking and worrying too much.

They will also help if asked when a person needs inspiration or illumination and when sitting examinations. The Air elementals, the Sylphs are as elusive as thoughts are in the human mind, and just as powerful.

Fire

The hot, darting light of the fire is home to the Fire Elementals, the Salamanders which to me appear like dragons in varying sizes, all moving swiftly with flickering tongues. In my youth, in the days of coal fires one could sit and watch the pictures in the grate of tiny Salamanders in their red-hot caves and shooting from coal to coal. Central heating may be more efficient but it lacks the beauty of a real fire!

The two main conditions where the Fire elementals can assist are those relating to circulation and problems with energy like continual tiredness. The heart and circulatory system keeps the body warm and also carries oxygen and nutrients as fuel for the cells in the body. Lack of energy, tiredness and complaints like ME or chronic fatigue syndrome are helped by the warm input of Salamanders, lending some of their energy to fire up the immune systems of the client. Fire elementals can also help with Sylphs when mental inspiration is needed as Fire needs Air to ensure its existence.

The gentle Fire energy of a candle may fire the imagination and aid a pathworking or visualisation. The Salamanders can aid the power of lasers doing surgery and can help the transformation of malignant cells into benign cells. This transforming aspect of Fire is often ignored but without it much of our food would be inedible and indigestible. We call on Fire elementals to burn out infected tissue, allowing healthy growth just as the stubble was burned to encourage the next year's corn harvest. Fire cauterises leaking blood vessels to reduce bruising and blood loss and the Salamanders can help fire up the will to recover from sickness so do not underestimate their potential for assisting with healing.

Water

The Water element relates to the emotional level of the subtle bodies and if we are aware of the amount of water in our physical bodies we will appreciate that the Water Elementals are often a great help with healing of emotions and certain physical ailments. Over many years sailors have reported seeing mermaids and other phenomena at sea. The Undines (or mermaids) would help the sailor in his lonely work far from friends and family just as they will help us too. The Undines of the different forms of Water may take on the attributes of the state of the water; snow flakes when the water is snow, tiny figures in many-hued raindrops, tumbling in waterfalls and white water or calm and gentle in a slowly flowing river or lake. Physical problems of the urinary and lymph systems can benefit from their help enabling the body to allow excess fluid and toxins to flow away. Similarly, the emotional conditions of depression, bereavement, relationship problems where it is necessary to let go and allow ourselves to go with the flow are all the province of the Undine.

With all these wonderful Helpers available to us to use with healing energy of the Earth and Cosmos, we can never really feel that we are working alone and it is most important that at the end of a healing session we bid our Helpers 'Hail and Farewell' as they return to 'Their fair and lovely Realms'.

Chapter 8

Using Goddess and God Energy

Whenever we are channelling healing from the Source of all life, health and joy we are, of course using the energies of the Goddess and the God who are the Source. However, it is sometimes helpful to call upon specific aspects of the Goddess or God as personified in particular deities.

If we are working with a client who feels the need to increase their assertiveness and reasoning abilities we may suggest an energy like that of Thor or Herne. Each healer will have their own pantheon of helping deities depending on their especial allegiance or path and those suggested here will reflect my personal usage. What is very useful to a healer is to draw up your own table or list of assisting Deities with the conditions which each helps to heal with you

My own list includes the following entries:

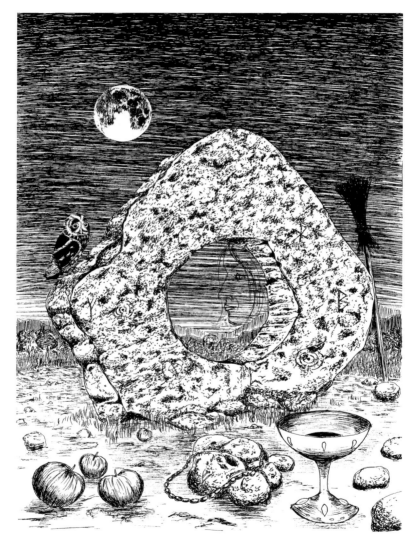

Goddess images

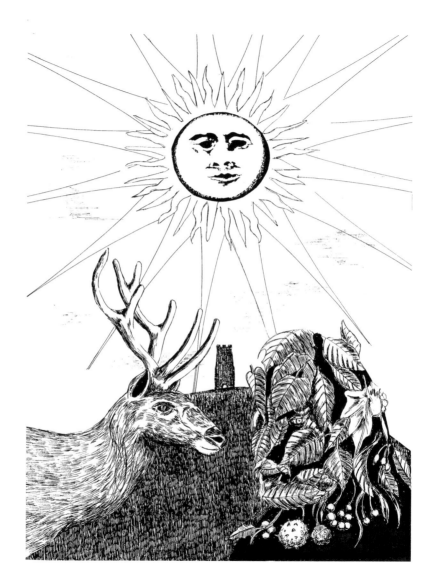

God images

Deity	Condition
Herne	Lack of assertiveness or direction in life.

Invocation

Great Herne, Lord of the Wildwood who can find your way in the darkest night or densest forest lend your strength of purpose and clear leadership to this person (or name) that he/she may feel your power and guidance at this time of need. I ask that You assist me now as the healing energy is offered to this person (or name) and as I do ask, so mote it be.

After the healing session is finished:

I thank you, Lord Herne for your help and assistance and I bid you Hail and Farewell.

Deity	Condition
Isis	Depression, life falling apart .

Invocation

Lady Isis, Queen of Heaven I ask for your help for (name) as he/she struggles to find his/her reasons for living and tries to put his/her life together again. Loving sister who searched the worlds to reclaim Osiris, who knows how to rebuild a being and a life, lend your hopefulness and caring loving

to the healing energy which we offer to (name).
Lady of Life, assist us now. So mote it be.

Afterwards:

I thank you, Lovely Queen for your help and
support and I bid you Hail and Farewell.

Deity	Condition
Brigid or Cerne	Infertility.
(depending on female or male client)	

Invocation

Lovely Lady Bridgid (or Great Lord Cernunnos) I
ask you to lend your fertile energy to (name) who
would wish to become a parent (or mother/father)
to a child of Earth. As the field is ploughed and
the seed sown to bring a fruitful harvest, assist
her/him in her/his endeavours to bring fruit to
her/his union with a beloved. Lovely Lady (Great
Lord), add your special power to this healing now
being offered. So mote it be.

Afterwards

I thank you, Blessed Lady (or Lord) for your help
and assistance and I bid you Hail and Farewell.

Often the invocation is one which comes to mind at the time and this may well be the best way for it to happen. Your own invocation from your centre of being and place of unconditional love may be only a feeling directed towards an aspect of the Goddess or the God, but if it is for the good of your client, it will be just as powerful as the most complicated invocation revealing all aspects of a particular Deity.

When looking at the different Pantheons and their relationships to healing, there appears to be only one Deity who has responsibility for healing without additional aspects. He is the Greek god Asclepias. All other deities have at least one other aspect to them although most of them can have healing as part of their attributes. Brigid or Bride is commonly thought of as predominantly healing energy but she is also the Goddess of Smithcraft, Fire, Poetry and Fertility.

Asclepias, the Greek god of healing was the son of Apollo and a lake nymph Coronis. While still pregnant with Asclepias, Coronis was killed by Artemis for being unfaithful to Apollo but Asclepias was rescued by his father and given into the care of Chiron. He learned the arts of medicine, surgery and healing and became so proficient that he could bring the dead back to life. This annoyed Hades who complained to Zeus. In order to maintain the balance of the world, Zeus killed Asclepias. His daughter Hygeia, the goddess of Health, and Hippocrates were among his followers. He is represented as a kindly man holding a staff around which a snake is entwined. The Roman equivalent to him is the God Aesculapius.

So to conclude my comments on using the energies of the Goddess and the God I turn my thoughts to Asclepias who is a god in a Pantheon with which I do not often work and I ask Him to assist us all as we endeavour to bring happiness, love and peace to all those who ask for healing. May His Healing Power enhance the energies we offer to those in need. So mote it be.

Chapter 9

Some other frequently used approaches to healing

(Dowsing, colour, crystals, sound)

As a healer, there are some other energies which can be used to create both an appropriate environment and also to assist in channelling the healing energy.

Dowsing can be used both diagnostically and as a focus for healing energy. It is usual when dowsing in this way to either use a pendulum or if you are especially able, just your hands. Using a pendulum has the advantage that the client can actually see the movement and any changes in direction. The way I use my pendulum is to ascertain the conditions of the chakras and to find any areas in the physical and subtle bodies of my client which are out of balance.

First, I run a check on the pendulum by asking it to show me its response for positive (or yes) and then for its response for negative (or no). I will also ask for it to move into neutral which is the position it will take while I ask my questions.

To work on the chakras, I will either hold the pendulum directly over the chakra or, if the client is upright I may place my left hand over or on the chakra, holding my pendulum in my right hand. I ask the question, Is this chakra in balance? . This may be spoken audibly or asked silently. If the response is positive I give thanks (ever so politely!) and move on to the next major chakra. If the response is negative, I put the pendulum in neutral and focus on healing, balancing energy into the chakra through the pendulum or through my left hand, I then ask the question again, repeating the procedure until the response is positive.

In order to scan over the physical body I ask the question Is this part of the body in balance? and move my left hand over or on the body watching for any changes in direction of the pendulum.

To check out the state of the different subtle bodies, the pendulum is held in the appropriate part of the aura and the name of the level given when the question is asked. Healing can be offered in the same way as chakra balancing.

The use of colour with healing is another field of study about which other books have been written. The ways in which I use it may be of interest here. First, my physical environment is painted and decorated with gentle greens and blues as these are colours of nature which are complementary for healing and which help to create a calm atmosphere. Secondly, when working on the chakras I find it beneficial to the client if I visualise the appropriate chakra colour to the one I am balancing.

People often see colour images or patches when they receive healing and these seem to relate to the chakric area which is receiving healing energy. Colour can also be visualised or a coloured silk placed on the client when using Elemental or specific Deity energies. When invoking Isis a deep, clear blue seems appropriate or maybe red for the energy of Fire. Here I would suggest that you listen to your own intuition; it isn't the actual colour which is important, what really matters is your intent. Colour does affect our human emotional conditions and as such is a helpful tool with healing.

My own work with crystals is limited to mainly personal use and to enhance the energy in my working environment. Occasionally, I will give a crystal to a client for them to hold while I am working and when choosing the stone I work entirely intuitively. Crystals which I use most are frequently rose quartz, aventurine, amethyst and obsidian. The colour of the crystal can also be relevant with chakra balancing and suggested co-relations are:

Base	Red	Garnet, ruby, bloodstone.
Sacral	Orange	Orange calcite, coral.
Solar plexus	Yellow	Citrine (light), amber.

Heart	Green	Aventurine, tourmaline.
Throat	Blue	Lapis lazuli, turquoise.
Third eye	Indigo/purple	Amethyst, Lapis lazuli.
Crown	White/violet	Clear quartz, Amethyst.

Place the crystal on the chakra (or hold it near) when offering healing. Other healers may use different crystals - find what works for you by trying them out and see what feels right, intuitively.

Sound is another area worthy of a study of its own. It is known that hearing is the last sense to be lost in the dying person and it can be sounds that will revive the comatose patient so it has a strong role to play in healing work.

At the simplest level, pleasant soft music or natural sounds produce a state of relaxation and well-being in most human beings. In the healing room, gentle background music can have this effect which will enhance the benefits which the healee will feel when receiving energy.

However, when used therapeutically by an experienced sound therapist, the vibrations of sound can produce profound effects. Long before anybody mentioned the New Age, shamans and other healers were using drums, rattles and bells to enhance their work and create altered states of consciousness. Mothers (and fathers too) have, since time began, used the human voice to calm and re-assure their young ones. Today, the hypnotherapist and counselling therapist also use their voices to calm, re-assure, encourage or confront their clients.

To gently talk the client through a relaxation exercise before offering healing can be helpful and re-assuring, especially if he/she is fearful or tense. The human voice is a powerful tool to use with healing energy and it is one which we all can use to enhance the work we do. It is not necessary to be able to sing like a professional, all you need to do is to murmur words of love and encouragement. You are the voice of the Source, the voice of the Goddess or the voice of the God. Blessed be!

Chapter 10

Some other complementary therapies and their relevance to the Pagan Healer

Aromatherapy

This usually involves massage as well as the use of essential oils for their beneficial effects. There is a strong link to Paganism as the aromatherapist is using the essence of the plant from which the oil originates. These oils would have been in use for many years before the term aromatherapist was coined. The ancient Greeks and Romans used oils, unguents and pomades gathered from different parts of the Empire and even before them the priests of the Egyptians and Babylonians dispensed aromatic oils for use as perfume, incense and medicines.

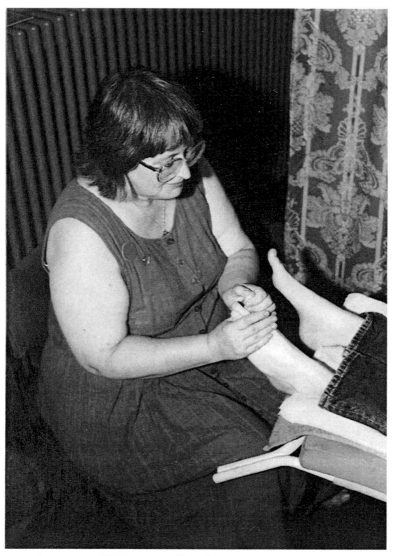

Giving a reflexology treatment

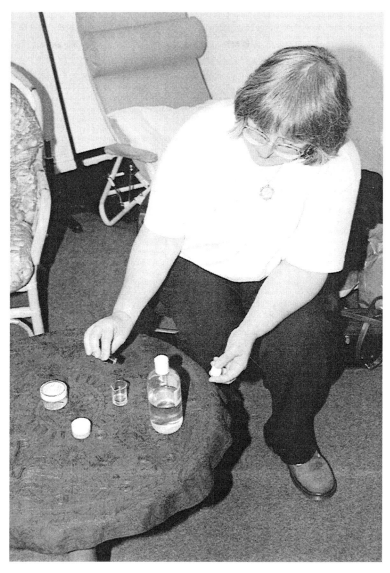

Preparing aromatherapy oils for massage

Bach Flower Remedies

These are prepared using organically grown flowers, spring water and sunlight. The energy of the plant is absorbed by the water under the sunlight and it is then preserved by the addition of brandy. This use of energy and natural ingredients seems to sit well with an it harm none and both these remedies and those prepared in the same way by other people seem very Pagan-friendly to me!

Counselling and Psychotherapy

The listening ear provided by therapists in these fields is an aspect of healing. Counsellors will not tell you what to do but will help you see yourself more clearly and using many different methods they will all hope that the client will become whole in their truest sense.

Herbalism

The old village herbalist ran the risk of being considered a witch but she (or he) was the only person available to help the sick. She knew the plants and fruits and used them for healing. Today the herbalist has many ingredients from other countries available to her/him but the basic aim of using plants and herbs to heal is the same.

Hypnotherapy/Past Life Regression

Just as the shaman used trance states to journey into other dimensions, so the hypnotherapist can enable the client to reach into the depths or heights of their own personalities by similar means. Past-life regression can also be achieved by the same technique and again can help deepen our understanding of ourselves. For the Pagan client this often reinforces the belief in and understanding of re-incarnation.

Massage

The healing power of touch as given in massage is a true, Pagan honouring of the body as a vehicle for the Goddess or God. When combined with the use of Essential oils, the client will feel relaxed and healthy after a treatment. Honour the Divine in your nearest and dearest by giving them a massage!

Reflexology

All the advantage of massage, combined with the accessibility of just using hands or feet. The accessing of the healing of unconditional love by the honouring of the feet is a moving healing experience. Highly recommended for all Pagans!

Reiki/Seichem

Reiki is an ancient healing art which was re-discovered by Dr Usui in the late 1800's and has been handed down to other practitioners via Reiki masters. Seichem is a development of Reiki incorporating the energies of Fire, Water and Air/Spirit. The use of the Elements makes this a most acceptable development of healing abilities for most Pagans and Reiki/Seichem can be incorporated into most healing modalities.

The Importance of Counselling in the Healing Process

When we consider or begin to offer healing, we have to be aware that the client may need healing in other parts of their body which may not be immediately obvious to us. When we offer healing, we offer it for it to be used in whatever way is best for the recipient. This may mean that the physical symptoms with which we are presented may only be one layer of many which cloak the real sickness of the person.

When healing is accepted the client may access those parts of their being which may distress them and activate an emotional response which needs attention. They may need assistance in coping with and understanding this re-action or they may need an empathetic person to support him/her and to be there for them.

The problem which we see is what could be called the reality of the middle self but another aspect of this may be in the client's Higher Self where it may manifest as avoidance or in the Lower Self where it becomes the shadow - that which is hidden, that which we do not want to see. By the use of counselling skills, the healer can help the client to take responsibility for their own healing and to face those hidden or avoided factors which caused the problem from the beginning. We can help the client acquire a healing attitude which does not allocate blame but which does accept responsibility.

The responsibility of the counsellor/healer is to maintain boundaries which enable the client to feel safe and to always be aware of the risk of letting the client spark off re-actions in the healer. This is not appropriate in the healing environment and the client should be referred to a qualified person if the healer feels that they may be likely to have this kind of re-action. The physical space in which healing is given needs to clean (psychically and physically). It is best if it is tidy and private with no telephone or door bells likely to disturb the healer or their client.

When a person arrives for a healing session or starts to react emotionally to a healing, she/he will be feeling very vulnerable and possibly distressed. At this point especially, the healer must be very aware and caring, responsive to the client's needs and comfort. During the session it must be ensured that the client feels safe at all times even or especially when they are beginning to face some of the deeply hidden areas of pain.

The healer is there for the client, listening solely to the client, not judging, accepting, responding genuinely but not rushing to comfort or make it feel better. In healing, as in many other therapies, it is often necessary to experience the deepest pain before true healing can commence. Sometimes it is only necessary to be present, allowing the silence, if that is O.K. with the client. In this stillness the deepest pain may be able to rise to the conscious level where it can be dealt with. This process can not be hurried, healing takes place at the speed dictated by the client and this may be a very slow pace indeed.

As healing commences in the subconscious, the presenting physical symptoms may change and here too they may seem to get worse before improving. If this occurs the healer will need to help the client appreciate what is happening.

When a client who has a life-threatening illness asks for healing, the importance of counselling in an appropriate way is seen again. The client may be in the final stages of a terminal disease like cancer or AIDS but can still benefit from empathetic counselling and healing. To give false hope would be unprofessional and unkind but to give supportive healing to the client and their carers is acceptable and appropriate.

Healing directed towards the emotional subtle body as well as the physical body can be very helpful. Using counselling skills combined with healing, the client can be healed on many levels enabling them to live each day at a time, taking responsibility for their own life. I feel that the importance of counselling in the healing process can not be emphasised too much and if possible, all potential professional healers should include a counselling unit in their training. The healing process is that in which the Higher Self or spirit accepts assistance from the energies of the earth or the cosmos, Goddess or God in order to return the body or subtle bodies of that person to optimal functioning i.e. HEALTH. Sometimes that assistance needs to be in the form of counselling alongside the healing as part of the whole process.

May the Goddess and the God endow all healers with good listening skills and the ability to only speak when necessary.

Blessed Be!

A Pathworking for Self-Healing

Sit yourself comfortably on a straight-backed chair with your feet firmly on the ground and your hands on your knees. Feel your head balanced on the top of your spine and try to keep your back as straight as is comfortable. Close your eyes.

Bring your focus down to your feet, curl and stretch your toes and then let all the tension go out of them. Do the same with first, your feet and then your ankles. Be aware that your ankles, feet and toes feel relaxed and soft.

Now bring your focus of attention up into the calf muscles of your legs, tighten these muscles and then let them go soft. Do this again if at first your muscles find it difficult to relax. Move up to your thigh muscles and repeat the tightening and relaxing, letting go of all tension until both of your legs fell soft and relaxed right down to your toes.

Bringing your attention now to your buttocks and abdomen, tighten up all these muscles which work so hard helping you to walk and protecting your abdominal organs. Now let them relax and allow

*all the tension to flow out of them. Move up to your
solar plexus and again tighten and relax these
muscles.*

*Just check downwards for any tension remaining
in your lower body and allow any tightness to flow
away. Feel your body from your solar plexus to
your toes to be soft and relaxed.*

*Continuing upwards, bring your focus to your rib-
cage which protects your heart and lungs. Feel the
tension in your upper back and shoulder area, in
your chest and lungs and allow it to leave your
body so that all this part of you also becomes soft
and relaxed.*

*Now allow this softness and relaxation to flow like
warmth down both of your arms to your very
finger-tips. Clench your fists and then relax and
gently shake them free of all tension.*

*The warmth begins to spread and to rise up your
neck, freeing it from stress and allowing it to relax
as the gentling flow engulfs your head and relaxes
your face and jaw.*

*Lovingly check your body for any last remaining
pockets of stress and allow them to leave. Take a
deep breath of pure, clean air, hold it for a few
moments in your body and then as you exhale feel
yourself settling gently down on your seat.*

*Now, I want you to picture yourself resting on the
grass and cool earth in a meadow. To one side of
the meadow a stream gurgles along on its way to*

the river, the sky above you is clear blue and the warmth of the sun is felt on your face as a gentle breeze ruffles your hair.

Rest in this place for a little while, feeling safe and happy. Look at the trees and plants, listen to the birds singing and the quiet sounds of the insects.

As you sit there clouds begin to build in the sky, not obscuring the sun but still shedding their raindrops on you and your meadow. A rainbow appears above you, brilliant and glowing with colour.

Looking at the innermost arc of colour you recognise the deep red which is the colour relating to your base chakra, draw some of the energy from the rainbow into your body, into your base chakra. Feel it's resonance with your physical body, feeding, nurturing and balancing it.

As your gaze moves outwards, pick up the glowing orange from the rainbow and absorb it into your sacral chakra, your sexual centre. Let it nurture the growth of your creativity. Feel its warmth and love.

Now you move to the yellow arc in the rainbow, it is the colour of dancing daffodils, daffodil yellow for your solar plexus. The happy feeling engulfs your chakra at your solar plexus, making you smile and appreciate the wonder of your body.

The colour of the next arc is a fresh grass green and as you look at it, it beams down into your heart chakra, bringing with it the love of the

85

Goddess, who wears the dress of green and the love of the God, the Green Man. Bask in their love, allow it to reach to the very centre of your being.

As you look at the rainbow again the clear blue of the next arc catches your attention. You draw it down to your throat chakra, feeling its clearing and cleaning energy freeing your vocal cords so that you want to sing. On your exhalation gently allow a soft sound to come from your throat and then fade away.

The outer rim of the rainbow is glowing now. The indigo, deep night-sky blue is focussing down onto your brow chakra. You see stars and planets, sparks of light in the velvety softness spread around you. Look in wonder and feel the reality of the heavens.

Lastly, the violet crown of the rainbow lifts you as it links to your crown chakra. Up you rise to reach the outermost limits of the cosmos, to combine with the energy of the Divine Source.

Slowly now, you begin to descend down the rainbow, returning to your place in the meadow. The rain stops and as the sun shines brightly the rainbow fades away. It leaves you with its blessings, you feel balanced and at ease with yourself on all levels of your existence. Recalling all the colours briefly, you relax on the firm earth and become aware again of the gentle breeze, the gurgling splashing of the stream and the healing warmth of the sun.

When you feel ready, become aware again of the chair on which you sit. Allow the meadow to fade but keep the feelings of balance, peace and serenity. Stretch your arms and legs and when you are fully aware of the room and this environment, open your eyes feeling refreshed and whole. Now stand up slowly and stamp both of your feet firmly on the ground before sitting down again. Have a drink of water or something to eat to fully ground yourself back into your body.

Case Histories

When one combines healing with both allopathic medicine and complementary therapies, it is always difficult to ascertain the efficiency of the treatment. However, healing does combine with and enhance other therapies by relaxing and re-assuring the patient thus enabling other treatments to function fully.

In my practice, it is rare for me to use only healing as I am qualified in reflexology, aromatherapy and counselling, but there are a few cases where none of the other therapies were used. I usually combine the healing with reflexology as more people find it acceptable to have their feet massaged and used to focus the healing energy.

Case History 1
Mrs. C. (aged 30) came to me five years ago for an aromatherapy massage. She presented symptoms of stress and gave her reason for coming as being in need of relaxation.

I used a simple oil blend of sweet almond oil and essential oil of lavender which is known for its relaxing and general therapeutic properties. When I had completed a full body massage and she was still relaxing on the couch, she started to tell me about her physical problems. She explained that she suffered from endometriosis, a fact which she had withheld when I took her medical details prior to the massage. This condition was, according to her consultant, making it difficult for her to conceive and causing pain during menstruation.

I had not attempted to "tune in" during the massage but had been aware of healing energy being absorbed by her when I had been working on her lower abdomen. I re-assured her that some healing had already taken place and offered to continue with more energy in-put. She accepted and I placed my hands on her abdomen again, channelling healing to her reproductive organs. Slowly she allowed the healing energy to begin flowing again and commented that the priest of her church may not approve of this treatment. I suggested that if she was concerned she could discuss it with him and offered her my card so that he could contact me if he so wished. As my hands began to cool I closed down the energy and ended the session. We made another appointment for massage two months hence and she went home.

Six weeks later she called to cancel the appointment for aromatherapy as she had just discovered that she was pregnant. Eighteen months later I met her and her son in the street and stopped for a chat. Shortly afterwards she telephoned to say that happily she was pregnant again. When I last heard from her, both of her sons were thriving. I did not receive any calls from the priest!!

Case History 2

As Mrs. S (aged 68 years) was house-bound, I had been asked by a relative to visit her at home and give her some healing. She was having difficulty walking as she had pains in her left leg which was also prone to swelling (oedema). Her doctor was suggesting that physiotherapy may help but there was a waiting list for appointments. She had been prescribed medication, but seemed reluctant to take it.

When I checked the aura around Mrs.S. there were cold patches at her neck, shoulders, hips and leg. She had quite a pronounced hump in her upper back but was adamant that it was not a problem. When checking the subtle bodies, I found a lot of disturbance in the emotional body.

After receiving healing, she reported that the leg seemed to have "drained up-wards" and was much more comfortable. She was also more up-right in her posture and said that she felt very relaxed and happy.

I made weekly visits for six weeks, during which time changes occurred in the family dynamics which relieved some of her concerns and she began to go out with a friend. She was able to stand much straighter and see where she was going, instead of looking at her feet all the time!

Case History 3

While working as a reflexologist at a health and psychic fair, I was approached by a girl with her leg in a plaster cast. She wanted to know whether healing would help her and I offered to give healing in order that she could find out for herself. In this case I simply put my hands around the cast in the aura and focussed healing into the broken tibia (shin-bone). She reported feeling great warmth and "a kind of tingling" in her leg as if it was healing.

Later, I heard from a mutual acquaintance that the doctors were amazed at her quick recovery and that full mobility was regained sooner than they expected.

Case History 4

When T. came to me she was in her early 40's and experiencing a time in her life when everything seemed to be going wrong. She had four sessions of healing fortnightly, during which I cleaned and filtered her subtle bodies, removing all negativity, at the same time I helped her to strengthen her belief in herself. I also taught her how to protect herself from external negativity and to build up her aura for herself.

Her life began to improve, work was available again and she felt physically much fitter. On an emotional level, she had more peace and self-esteem and assured me that it was to the healing that she attributed her recovery.

Case History 5

When my grandson was born he had a very difficult delivery and his first experience of life outside the womb was a stomach wash-out. Following this he cried continuously when not feeding or sleeping and nobody could pacify him. When I visited him on the day after his birth, my son (a fervent Christian!) almost threw Tom at me with the words, "See what you can do with him".

As I held the tiny, distressed child, I placed my hand on his abdomen and chest, channelling healing energy. Almost at once, he stopped crying and looked at me in silent gratitude. My son asked what magic I was using and I asked him whether it was important! He agreed that if his son was happy and quiet the it was O.K. with him, too.

Some months later Thomas developed meningitis which was only just diagnosed in time for appropriate treatment to be given. The church held a healing session around his hospital cot and I sent absent healing from home as well as giving "hands on" when I saw him. Together with drugs and good nursing care, these healing energies enabled him to be considered fit enough to go home after only 5 days in hospital.

Conclusion

If you have read this book up to here, then my suggestion is that now you start to practise some of the exercises contained in it. This is intended as a guide to doing , not just a book to be read and then left on the shelf. Take your own natural, Goddess-God given abilities and use them. If you feel you need further teaching or guidance - ask for it and if you feel drawn to be a professional healer, please make sure that you do receive adequate training and insurance.

I invite Bridget, Goddess of Healing to guide and lead all who read this book, onwards in their journey of discovery of their own innate healing abilities. May She light your Paths with Her Fire and may you always recognise and honour the Divine in Yourself.

Blessed be,

Liz Joan

Further Reading

The Complete Book of Family Aromatherapy,
  Joan Radford

Channelling for Everyone, Tony Neate

The Reflexology and Colour Therapy Workbook,
  Pauline Wills

Culpepper's Colour Herbal

Hands of Light, Barbara Ann Brennan

Light Emerging, Barbara Ann Brennan

Healing with Crystals, Jacquie Burgess

The Psychology of Healing, Murray Hope

The Tibetan Book of Living and Dying

How to Meditate, Laurence Le Shan

*Chaos International No. 21, Magic for Healing - A
  Shamanic Perspective*, Phil Hine

Reiki and Other Rays of Touch Healing,
  Kathleen Milner

Magic Without Peers, Ariadne Rainbird and David
  Rankine

Index

A selection from over 100 other titles published by Capall Bann. A free detailed catalogue is available on request.

The Journey Home   by Chris Thomas

Channelled writings have had their relevance and many are of great importance to humankind at this time of transition. However, none have attempted to tackle our basic, fundamental longing for answers the age-old questions: Who are we? Why are we here? Are we alone? What relationship does Earth and its multitude of lifeforms have to themselves and to the universe as a whole? The answers to many of these questions have been available since mankind appeared on the planet, but over the centuries they have become hidden by personal interests and clouded by repetition and dogma. As humankind undergoes a vast shift in consciousness, the underlying reasons for humankind's existence have to be rediscovered and put into their proper perspective. This book brings these issues into a sharper focus and sheds light into some of the darker corners. Gone are the dark days of Karmic re-cycling and suffering; we have reached the time of the birth of a new human existence so far removed from human experience that most have not yet recognised its coming.

ISBN 186163 041 7   **£7.95**

Working With The Merlin - Healing People and Planet   by Geoff Hughes

The Merlin is a guardian of this planet, together with many others and is acting on behalf of other unseen guardians, seeking mankind's help in restoring harmony to all here. This book is about the Merlin and his teachings in the 1980's and 1990's. The Merlin has awoken, for now is his time to move about the Land again to bring healing to the peoples, the lands and the earth. The writer is, like many others, on a Quest. The Quest for knowledge, to Know, to search for a meaning of life and what things are all about. The answers which came through are stunning, sometimes shocking, often controversial. This book is about aspects of this work, carefully graded to take the aspiring student through the first principles and onward into the realms of having the ability to make direct contact with the Forces of the Cosmos. Cutting through the mountains of superstition and man-made rules to find the simplicity and purity of our natural heritage of direct contact with the Unseen Worlds.

ISBN 186163 0018   £10.95

The Healing Book   by Chris Thomas & Diane Baker

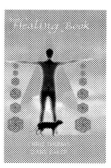

This book is for those who wish to heal. The book starts at the beginning of the healing process with simple, easily followed exercises which can begin to unlock the healing potential which is inherent in all of us. Nobody needs to feel left out of these abilities. Whatever level of experience you have of healing, this book explains in simple uncomplicated language that does not use mysticism or any form of ritual. These methods apply equally to humans and to animals. If you do not have any experience of giving healing, but would like to learn, this book can set you on that path. If you already work as a healer, in whatever capacity, and would like to explore your greater potential, this book is also for you.

ISBN 186163 053 0   £8.95

The Face of the Deep - Healing Body and Soul

by Penny Allen

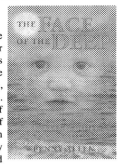

We cannot truly heal our bodies or minds without recognising the needs of the soul. The healing process appears magical or miraculous only when we do not understand the inner workings behind life. Outer and inner are inseparable. Ancient gods share their names with the planets and their influences with colours, music, numbers and chakras, the energy wheels within our bodies. Penny Allen has a background as a journalist and a teacher of literature as well as twenty years of experience as a teacher of meditation and as a healer, counsellor and astrologer. Drawing on mythology, she leads us on a fascinating journey of discovery showing how the soul is linked to the body and mind and concluding that, if we are to heal ourselves and our environment, we must align ourselves once again to the universe of which we are part. ISBN 186163 0409 £9.95

Psychic Self Defence - Real Solutions by Jan Brodie

How to recognise a psychic attack & how to handle it? This book concentrates on a commonsense approach to problems including interviews describing how people have dealt with attacks. Practical information, based on real experiences, is given on a range of protective & self development measures:- Summoning a guardian. Banishing 'evil' influences, Holding your own in the Otherworlds/Astral levels. Protective amulets & talismans, Strengthening the aura, Increasing self-confidence in magical work & visualisation, Psychic attack - What it is and is not, Elemental Spirits of Nature, Guardian Spirits, the Aura, the Astral Levels, the Psychic Vampire, the Realm of Faerie, Ghosts, Psychic Attack Through Willpower & the Evil Eye.
ISBN 1898307 36 9   £8.95

Crystal Doorways by Sue & Simon Lilly

This is not yet another volume telling you everything you wanted to know about crystals. It focuses on a very particular system of using crystals and colour to bring about changes in your consciousness and an increasing understanding of the energy world around us. The idea of using crystals placed on and around the body has been known for a long time, but most layouts required a vast number of large and expensive crystals or an honours degree in geometry to work them out. Developed as a result of running many courses, 'Crystal Doorways' gives a clear, immediately understandable, system of "energy nets" using small, easily obtainable crystals. These energy nets are simple, usually only requiring small tumbled stones, but they can be extremely powerful. Each net is illustrated and described in full, with what stones to use, where to place them, potential uses and background information.
ISBN 1898307 98 9   £11.95   **R97**   Illustrated

Healing Stones   by Sue Phillips

There is an increasing interest in crystals, from collectors, magicians and healers, with correspondingly increased pressure on our earth's precious resources. Healing stones sets out a method that works on the same principles as crystal healing, but makes use of stones and pebbles that can be found lying around almost anywhere. Here is a chance to learn what any child knows instinctively - stones are magical.

Healing Homes by Jennifer Dent

"What is home? Home is the place where we define our boundaries and express our inner selves. A place to which we belong. A place to be uniquely ourselves. a place of security, of connection, of renewal, of healing, a place to dream. Home, they say, is where the heart is".
"What is healing? At the most basic level it is to bring back into balance that which has become unbalanced." 'Healing Homes' is a book to inspire home-makers everywhere. A home should not just look good, it should nurture our inner needs. This is the accumulation of years of interest in, study and practical implementation of all the many aspects that go into the creation of a truly healing home. It introduces the ways in which colour and shape, light and sound, patterns, plants, herbs, crystals, music and the cycles of nature can be blended. Topics covered include: Healing, Earth energies, Cycles, Symbols, Shape, Light, Colour, Sound, Music, Feng Shui, Air, Earth, Fire, Water, Fragrance, Plants, Flowers, Crystals, Flower remedies, Homeopathy, Aromatherapy, Herbs and Gardens. A home filled with love, beauty and a healing ambience, sets the scene for you to lead a healthy and fulfiling life. This is very much a practical book which allows the reader to make empowered choices, leading to the creation of a personally healing home. ISBN 1898307 466   £9.95

Personal Power - Sacred Energies of Mind, Body and Spirit
by Anna Franklin

Personal Power is a course in personal and spiritual growth which was developed over twelve years in the Hearth of Arianrhod's Foundation Circle. Each chapter takes the form of a discussion of the energies and principles involved, followed by exercises and pathworkings which will help you develop the skills and thought patterns necessary to heal your life and centre you on your spiritual path. It covers the relationship between the mind, the body and the spirit, explored through the aura, the chakras, personal holistic healing and channelling energies and goes on to show how these powers are the foundation for healing, magic and psychic development.
ISBN 186161 0301

Magick Without Peers by Ariadne Rainbird & David Rankine
A Course in Progressive Witchcraft for the Solitary Practitioner

This is a book about Progressive Witchcraft which the authors see as being more eclectic and universal than Alexandrian and Gardnerian Wicca. Witchcraft is composed of three main elements - Magic, Mysticism and Religion - each treated in depth, and integrated in this excellent, practical book. Witchcraft contains elements of Shamanism and this book includes techniques such as dance, breathing techniques and the use of sacred herbs to explore other states of consciousness. Techniques and teaching from many different countries and cultures are integrated and used to great effect, drawn from the courses and teachings carried out by the authors. The book gives a solid grounding in personal magical work, aimed primarily at the sole practitioner, though members of groups will also benefit from the teachings given. ISBN 1898307 99 7 £12.95

Self Enlightenment   by Mayan O'Brien

Are you on a quest for truth, knowledge and wisdom? If so, this book will be a guide and a stepping stone for you. *Self Enlightenment* is full of practical advice on many areas of life. It discusses meditation, visualisation, the aura, examining our lives, creating a mind map, using astrology, the University of the solar System (a guided visualisation), the Tree of Life, health and herbs and how to organise a retreat for yourself. This book can be seen as a beacon to illuminate your way. ISBN 186163 0484   £9.95

FREE DETAILED CATALOGUE

A detailed illustrated catalogue is available on request, SAE or International Postal Coupon appreciated. **Titles can be ordered direct from Capall Bann, post free in the UK** (cheque or PO with order) or from good bookshops and specialist outlets. Titles currently available include:

Animals, Mind Body Spirit & Folklore
Angels and Goddesses - Celtic Christianity & Paganism by Michael Howard
Arthur - The Legend Unveiled by C Johnson & E Lung
Auguries and Omens - The Magical Lore of Birds by Yvonne Aburrow
Book of the Veil The by Peter Paddon
Caer Sidhe - Celtic Astrology and Astronomy by Michael Bayley
Call of the Horned Piper by Nigel Jackson
Cats' Company by Ann Walker
Celtic Lore & Druidic Ritual by Rhiannon Ryall
Compleat Vampyre - The Vampyre Shaman: Werewolves & Witchery by Nigel Jackson
Crystal Clear - A Guide to Quartz Crystal by Jennifer Dent
Earth Dance - A Year of Pagan Rituals by Jan Brodie
Earth Harmony - Places of Power, Holiness and Healing by Nigel Pennick
Earth Magic by Margaret McArthur
Enchanted Forest - The Magical Lore of Trees by Yvonne Aburrow
Familiars - Animal Powers of Britain by Anna Franklin
Healing Homes by Jennifer Dent
Herbcraft - Shamanic & Ritual Use of Herbs by Susan Lavender & Anna Franklin
In Search of Herne the Hunter by Eric Fitch
Magical Incenses and Perfumes by Jan Brodie
Magical Lore of Cats by Marion Davies
Magical Lore of Herbs by Marion Davies
Masks of Misrule - The Horned God & His Cult in Europe by Nigel Jackson
Mysteries of the Runes by Michael Howard
Patchwork of Magic by Julia Day
Psychic Self Defence - Real Solutions by Jan Brodie
Runic Astrology by Nigel Pennick
Sacred Animals by Gordon MacLellan
Sacred Grove - The Mysteries of the Forest by Yvonne Aburrow
Sacred Geometry   by Nigel Pennick
Sacred Lore of Horses The by Marion Davies
Sacred Ring - Pagan Origins British Folk Festivals & Customs by Michael Howard
Seasonal Magic - Diary of a Village Witch by Paddy Slade
Secret Places of the Goddess by Philip Heselton
Talking to the Earth by Gordon Maclellan
Taming the Wolf - Full Moon Meditations by Steve Hounsome
The Goddess Year by Nigel Pennick & Helen Field
West Country Wicca by Rhiannon Ryall

Capall Bann is owned and run by people actively involved in many of the areas in which we publish. Our list is expanding rapidly so do contact us for details on the latest releases.

Capall Bann Publishing, Freshfields, Chieveley, Berks, RG20 8TF